The Ultimate Ketogenic Air Fryer Recipe Collection

Quick and Easy Ketogenic Air Fryer Recipes to Boost Your Metabolism

Michael Clark

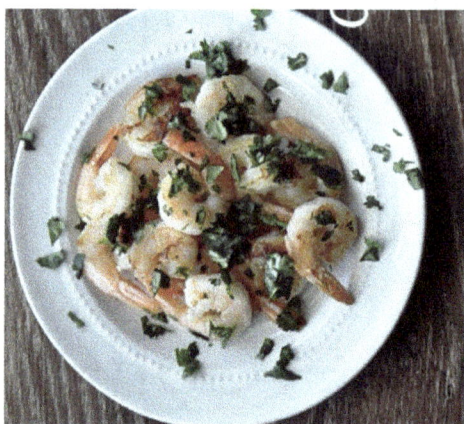

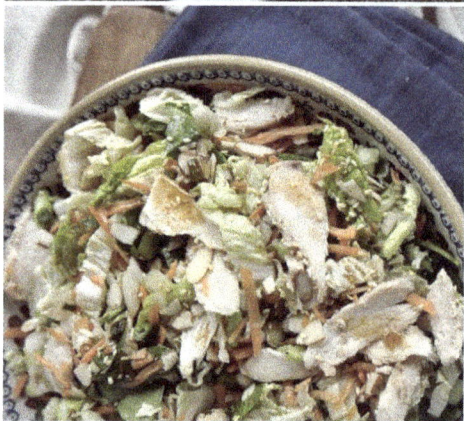

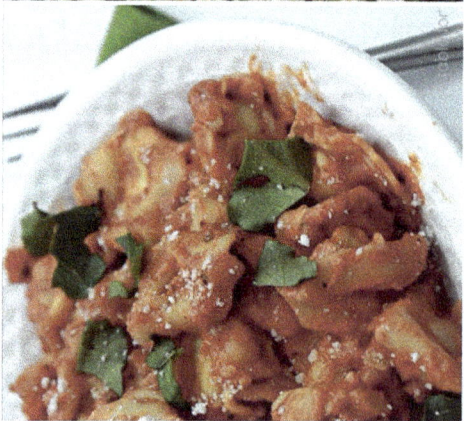

advice. The content within this book has been derived from various sources. Please consult a licensed professional before attempting any techniques outlined in this book.

By reading this document, the reader agrees that under no circumstances is the author responsible for any losses, direct or indirect, which are incurred as a result of the use of information contained within this document, including, but not limited to, — errors, omissions, or inaccuracies.

Table of Contents

Pork and Asparagus

Preparation time: 5 minutes

Cooking time: 35 minutes

Servings: 4

Ingredients:

- pounds pork loin, boneless and cubed
- ¾ cup beef stock
- tablespoons olive oil
- tablespoons keto tomato sauce
- 1 pound asparagus, trimmed and halved
- ½ tablespoon oregano, chopped Salt and black pepper to the taste

Directions:

1. Heat up a pan that fits your air fryer with the oil over medium heat, add the pork, toss and brown for 5 minutes. Add the rest of the ingredients, toss a bit, put the pan in the fryer and cook at 380 degrees F for 30 minutes. Divide everything between plates and serve.

Nutrition: calories 287, fat 13, fiber 4, carbs 6, protein 18

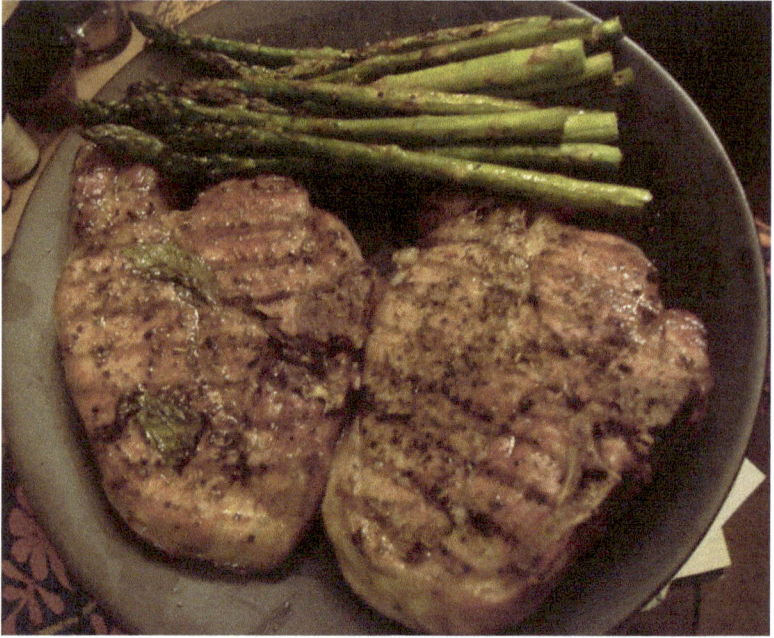

Wrapped Pork

Prep time: 20 minutes

Cooking time: 16 minutes

Servings: 2

Ingredients:

- 8 oz pork tenderloin
- 4 bacon slices
- ½ teaspoon salt
- 1 teaspoon olive oil
- ½ teaspoon chili powder

Directions:

1. Sprinkle the pork tenderloin with salt and chili powder. Then wrap it in the bacon slices and sprinkle with olive oil. Secure the bacon with toothpicks if needed. After this, preheat the air fryer to 375F. Put the wrapped pork tenderloin in the air fryer and cook it for 7 minutes. After this, carefully flip the meat on another side and cook it for 9 minutes more. When the meat is cooked,

remove the toothpicks from it (if the toothpicks were used) and slice the meat.

Nutrition: calories 390, fat 22.3, fiber 0.2, carbs 0.9, protein 43.8

Cinnamon Ghee Pork Chops

Preparation time: 5 minutes

Cooking time: 35 minutes

Servings: 4

Ingredients:

- 4 pork chops, bone-in
- A pinch of salt and black pepper 2 and ½ tablespoons ghee, melted
- ½ teaspoon chipotle chili powder
- ½ teaspoon cinnamon powder
- ½ teaspoon garlic powder
- ½ teaspoon allspice
- 1 teaspoon coconut sugar

Directions:

1. Rub the pork chops with all the other ingredients, put them in your air fryer's basket and cook at 380 degrees F for 35 minutes. Divide the chops between plates and serve with a side salad.

Nutrition: calories 287, fat 14, fiber 4, carbs 7, protein 18

Creamy Pork Chops

Prep time: 15 minutes

Cooking time: 10 minutes

Servings: 4

Ingredients:

- 2 pork chops
- ¼ cup coconut flakes
- 3 tablespoons almond flour
- ½ teaspoon salt
- ½ teaspoon dried parsley
- 1 egg, beaten
- 1 tablespoon heavy cream
- 1 teaspoon butter, melted

Directions:

1.   Cut every pork chops into 2 chops. Then sprinkle them with salt and dried parsley. After this, in the mixing bowl mix up coconut flakes and almond flour. In the separated bowl mix up egg, heavy cream, and melted

butter. Coat the pork chops in the almond flour mixture and them dip in the egg mixture. Repeat the same steps one more time. Then coat the pork chops in the remaining almond flour mixture. Place the meat in the air fryer basket. Cook the pork chops for 10 minutes at 400F. Flip them on another side after 5 minutes of cooking.

Nutrition: calories 303, fat 25.6, fiber 2.7, carbs 5.5, protein 15.1

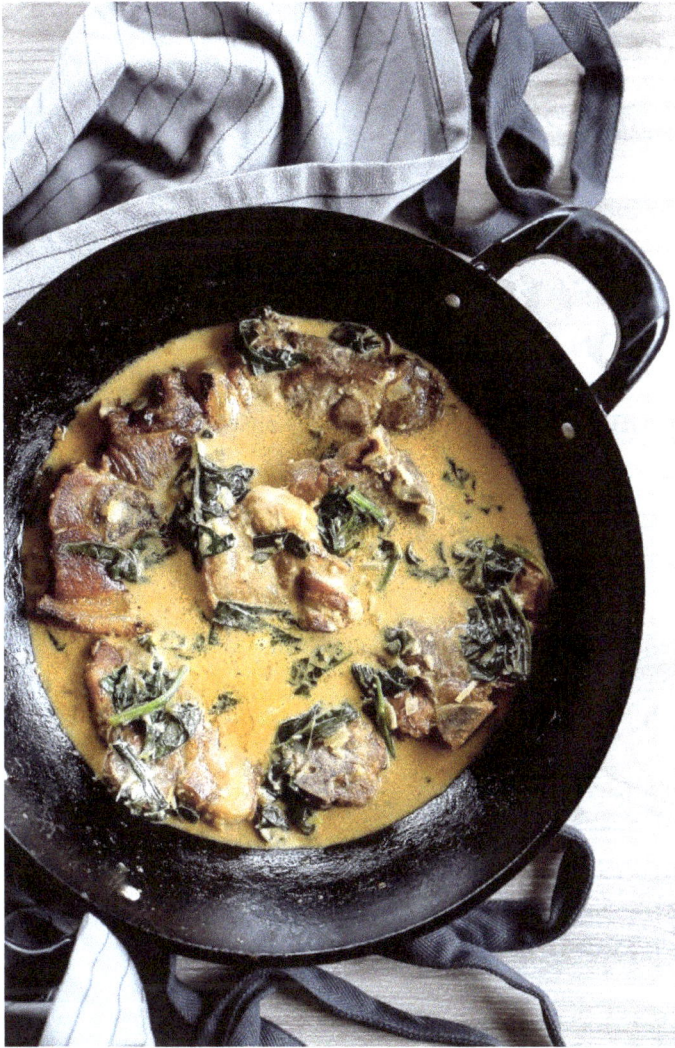

Shoulder

Prep time: 20 minutes

Cooking time: 20 minutes

Servings: 4

Ingredients:

- 1-pound pork shoulder, boneless
- 3 spring onions, chopped
- 1 teaspoon dried dill
- 1 teaspoon keto tomato sauce
- 1 tablespoon water
- 1 teaspoon salt
- 2 tablespoons sesame oil
- 1 teaspoon ground black pepper
- ½ teaspoon garlic powder

Directions:

1.   In the shallow bowl mix up salt, ground black pepper, and garlic powder. Then add dried dill. Sprinkle

the pork shoulder with a spice mixture from each side. Then in the separated bowl, mix up tomato sauce, water, and sesame oil. Brush the meat with the tomato mixture. Then place it on the foil. Add spring onions. Wrap the pork shoulder. Preheat the air fryer to 395F. Put the wrapped pork shoulder in the air fryer basket and cook it for 20 minutes. Let the cooked meat rest for 5-10 minutes and then discard the foil.

Nutrition: calories 401, fat 31.1, fiber 0.5, carbs 2.3, protein 26.8

Cocoa Ribs

Preparation time: 5 minutes

Cooking time: 45 minutes

Servings: 4

Ingredients:

- 2 tablespoons cocoa powder

- ½ teaspoon cinnamon powder

- ½ teaspoon chili powder

- 1 tablespoon coriander, chopped

- ½ teaspoon cumin, ground 2 racks of ribs

- A pinch of salt and black pepper Cooking spray

Directions:

1.   Grease the ribs with the cooking spray, mix with the other ingredients and rub very well. Put the ribs in your air fryer's basket and cook at 390 degrees F for 45 minutes. Divide between plates and serve with a side salad.

Nutrition: calories 284, fat 14, fiber 5, carbs 7, protein 20

Beef and Thyme Cabbage Mix

Preparation time: 5 minutes

Cooking time: 25 minutes

Servings: 4

Ingredients:

• pounds beef, cubed

• ½ pound bacon, chopped 2 shallots, chopped

• 1 napa cabbage, shredded 2 garlic cloves, minced

• A pinch of salt and black pepper 2 tablespoons olive oil

• 1 teaspoon thyme, dried 1 cup beef stock

Directions:

1. Heat up a pan that fits the air fryer with the oil over medium-high heat, add the beef and brown for 3 minutes. Add the bacon, shallots and garlic and cook for 2 minutes more. Add the rest of the ingredients, toss, put the pan in the air fryer and cook at 390 degrees F for 20 minutes. Divide between plates and serve.

Nutrition: calories 284, fat 14, fiber 2, carbs 6, protein 19

Butter Beef

Prep time: 10 minutes

Cooking time: 10 minutes

Servings: 4

Ingredients:

- 4 beef steaks (3 oz each steak)
- 4 tablespoons butter, softened
- 1 teaspoon ground black pepper
- ½ teaspoon salt

Directions:

1. In the shallow bowl mix up softened butter, ground black pepper, and salt. Then brush the beef steaks with the butter mixture from each side. Preheat the air fryer to 400F. Put the butter steaks in the air fryer and cook them for 5 minutes from each side.

Nutrition: calories 261, fat 16.8, fiber 0.1 carbs 0.4, protein 26

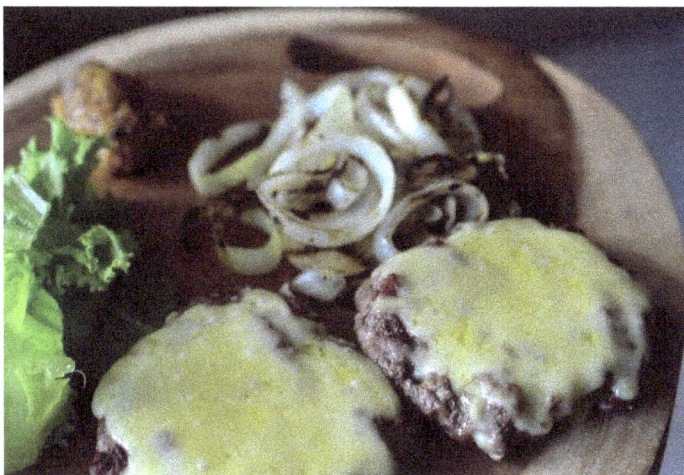

Almond Meatloaf

Preparation time: 5 minutes

Cooking time: 25 minutes

Servings: 4

Ingredients:

• 1 pound beef meat, ground 3 tablespoons almond meal Cooking spray

• 1 egg, whisked

• Salt and black pepper to the taste 1 tablespoon parsley, chopped

• 1 tablespoon oregano, chopped 2 spring onions, chopped

Directions:

1. In a bowl, mix all the ingredients except the cooking spray, stir well and put in a loaf pan that fits the air fryer. Put the pan in the fryer and cook at 390 degrees F for 25 minutes. Slice and serve hot.

Nutrition: calories 284, fat 14, fiber 3, carbs 6, protein 18

Nutmeg Pork Cutlets

Prep time: 10 minutes

Cooking time: 11 minutes

Servings: 3

Ingredients:

- 3 pork cutlets (3 oz each cutlet)
- 2 oz Parmesan, grated
- 1 tablespoon almond flour
- ½ teaspoon chili powder
- ¼ teaspoon ground nutmeg
- 1 teaspoon sesame oil
- 1 teaspoon lemon juice
- 1 egg, beaten

Directions:

1.   In the mixing bowl mix up Parmesan, almond flour, chili powder, and ground nutmeg. In the separated bowl mix up lemon juice and egg. After this, dip the pork cutlets in the egg mixture and then coat in the Parmesan

mixture. Sprinkle every coated cutlet with sesame oil. Preheat the air fryer to 400F. Place the pork cutlets in the air fryer basket and cook them for 6 minutes. Then carefully flip them on another side and cook for 5 minutes more.

Nutrition: calories 423, fat 33, fiber 1.2, carbs 3.2, protein 29.1

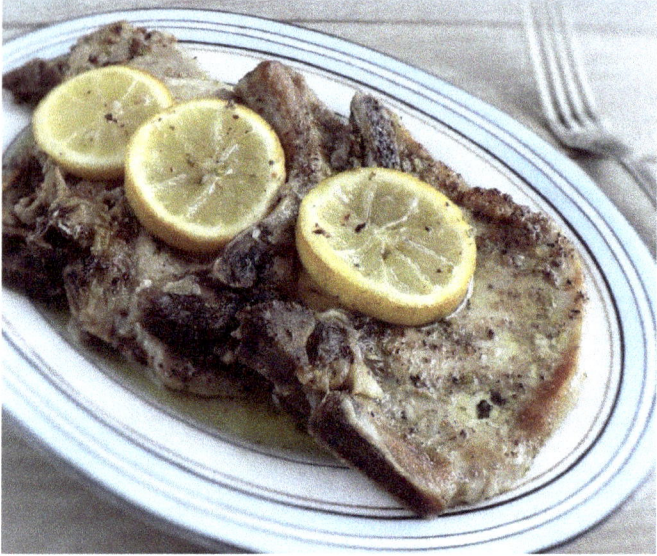

Chocolate and Avocado Cream

Preparation time: 5 minutes

Cooking time: 20 minutes

Servings: 4

Ingredients:

- avocados, peeled, pitted and mashed 3 tablespoons chocolate, melted

- 4 tablespoons erythritol

- 3 tablespoons cream cheese, soft

Directions:

1. In a pan that fits the air fryer, combine all the ingredients, whisk, put the pan in the fryer and cook at 340 degrees F for 20 minutes. Divide into bowls and serve cold.

Nutrition: calories 200, fat 6, fiber 2, carbs 4, protein 5

Sweet Coconut Cream Pie

Prep time: 15 minutes

Cooking time: 25 minutes

Servings: 4

Ingredients:

- 4 tablespoons coconut cream

- 1 teaspoon baking powder

- 1 teaspoon apple cider vinegar

- 1 egg, beaten

- ¼ cup coconut flakes

- 1 teaspoon vanilla extract

- ½ cup coconut flour

- 4 teaspoons Splenda

- 1 teaspoon xanthan gum

- Cooking spray

Directions:

1.   Put all liquid ingredients in the bowl: coconut cream, apple cider vinegar, egg, and vanilla extract. Stir the liquid until homogenous and add baking powder, coconut flakes, coconut flour, Splenda, and xanthan gum. Stir the ingredients until you get the smooth texture of the batter. Spray the air fryer cake mold with cooking spray. Pour the batter in the cake mold.

2.   Preheat the air fryer to 330F. Put the cake mold in the air fryer basket and cook it for 25 minutes. Then cool the cooked pie completely and remove it from the cake mold. Cut the cooked pie into servings.

Nutrition: calories 110, fat 6.6, fiber 3.9, carbs 9.9, protein 2.1

Cocoa Bombs

Preparation time: 5 minutes

Cooking time: 8 minutes

Servings: 12

Ingredients:

- 2 cups macadamia nuts, chopped 4 tablespoons coconut oil, melted 1 teaspoon vanilla extract

- ¼ cup cocoa powder 1/3 cup swerve

Directions:

1. In a bowl, mix all the ingredients and whisk well. Shape medium balls out of this mix, place them in your air fryer and cook at 300 degrees F for 8 minutes. Serve cold.

Nutrition: calories 120, fat 12, fiber 1, carbs 2, protein 1

Cinnamon Squash Pie

Prep time: 15 minutes

Cooking time: 35 minutes

Servings: 6

Ingredients:

- 2 tablespoons Splenda
- 1 tablespoon Erythritol
- 5 eggs, beaten
- 4 tablespoons coconut flakes
- ¼ cup heavy cream
- 1 teaspoon vanilla extract
- 1 teaspoon butter
- ¼ teaspoon ground cinnamon
- 4 oz Kabocha squash, peeled

Directions:

1.   Grate the Kabocha squash. Then grease the baking mold with butter and put the grated Kabocha squash

inside. In the mixing bowl mix up Splenda, Erythritol, coconut flakes, heavy cream, vanilla extract, and ground cinnamon. Then pour the liquid over the Kabocha squash. Stir the mixture gently with the help of the fork. Then preheat the air fryer to 365F. Put the mold with pie in the air fryer and cook it for 35 minutes. Cool the cooked pie to the room temperature and cut into the servings.

Nutrition: calories 116, fat 7.2, fiber 0.6, carbs 6.7, protein 5.1

Avocado Cake

Preparation time: 10 minutes

Cooking time: 30 minutes

Servings: 4

Ingredients:

- 4 ounces raspberries
- avocados, peeled, pitted and mashed 1 cup almonds flour
- teaspoons baking powder 1 cup swerve
- tablespoons butter, melted 4 eggs, whisked

Directions:

1. In a bowl, mix all the ingredients, toss, pour this into a cake pan that fits the air fryer after you've lined it with parchment paper, put the pan in the fryer and cook at 340 degrees F for 30 minutes. Leave the cake to cool down, slice and serve.

Nutrition: calories 193, fat 4, fiber 2, carbs 5, protein 5

Blueberry Cookies

Prep time: 10 minutes

Cooking time: 30 minutes

Servings: 2

Ingredients:

- 3 oz blueberries
- ½ teaspoon avocado oil

Directions:

1.   Put the blueberries in the blender and grind them until smooth. Then line the air fryer basket with baking paper. Brush it with the avocado oil. After this, pour the blended blueberries on the prepared baking paper and flatten it in one layer with the help of the spatula. Cook the blueberry leather for 30 minutes at 300F. Cut into cookies and serve.

Nutrition: calories 26, fat 0.3, fiber 1.1, carbs 6.2, protein 0.3

Strawberry Cups

Preparation time: 5 minutes

Cooking time: 10 minutes

Servings: 8

Ingredients:

- 16 strawberries, halved

- 2 tablespoons coconut oil

- 2 cups chocolate chips, melted

Directions:

1. In a pan that fits your air fryer, mix the strawberries with the oil and the melted chocolate chips, toss gently, put the pan in the air fryer and cook at 340 degrees F for 10 minutes. Divide into cups and serve cold.

Nutrition: calories 162, fat 5, fiber 3, carbs 5, protein 6

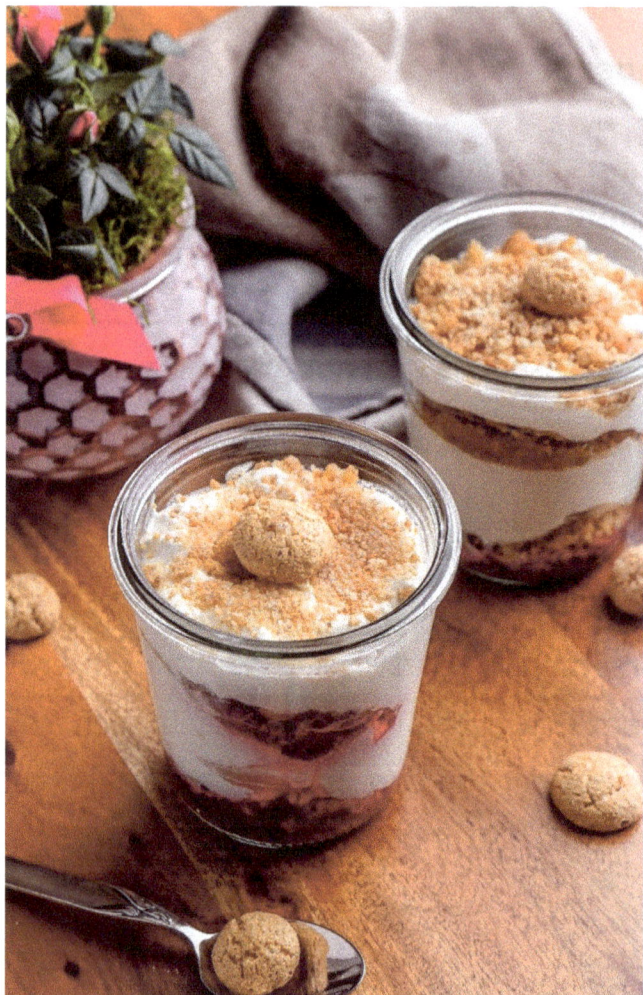

Cardamom Squares

Prep time: 15 minutes

Cooking time: 20 minutes

Servings: 4

Ingredients:

- 4 tablespoons peanut butter

- 1 tablespoon peanut, chopped

- 1 teaspoon vanilla extract

- ½ cup coconut flour

- 1 tablespoon Erythritol

- ½ teaspoon ground cardamom

Directions:

1.   Put the peanut butter and peanut in the bowl. Add vanilla extract, coconut flour, and ground cardamom. Then add Erythritol and stir the mixture until homogenous. Preheat the air fryer to 330F. Line the air fryer basket with baking paper and pour the peanut butter mixture over it. Flatten it gently and cook for 20

minutes. Then remove the cooked mixture from the air fryer and cool it completely. Cut the dessert into the squares.

Nutrition: calories 181, fat 11.7, fiber 7.2, carbs 12.8, protein 7.6

Strawberry Cake

Preparation time: 10 minutes

Cooking time: 35 minutes

Servings: 6

Ingredients:

- 1 pound strawberries, chopped 1 cup cream cheese, soft
- ¼ cup swerve
- 1 tablespoon lime juice 1 egg, whisked
- 1 teaspoon vanilla extract
- 3 tablespoons coconut oil, melted 1 cup almond flour
- 2 teaspoons baking powder

Directions:

1. In a bowl, mix all the ingredients, stir well and pour this into a cake pan lined with parchment paper. Put the pan in the air fryer, cook at 350 degrees F for 35 minutes, cool down, slice and serve.

Nutrition: calories 200, fat 6, fiber 2, carbs 4, protein 6

Butter Crumble

Prep time: 20 minutes

Cooking time: 25 minutes

Servings: 4

Ingredients:

- ½ cup coconut flour

- 2 tablespoons butter, softened

- 2 tablespoon Erythritol

- 3 oz peanuts, crushed

- 1 tablespoon cream cheese

- 1 teaspoon baking powder

- ½ teaspoon lemon juice

Directions:

1.   In the mixing bowl mix up coconut flour, butter, Erythritol, baking powder, and lemon juice. Stir the mixture until homogenous. Then place it in the freezer for 10 minutes. Meanwhile, mix up peanuts and cream cheese. Grate the frozen dough. Line the air fryer mold

with baking paper. Then put ½ of grated dough in the mold and flatten it. Top it with cream cheese mixture. Then put remaining grated dough over the cream cheese mixture. Place the mold with the crumble in the air fryer and cook it for 25 minutes at 330F.

Nutrition: calories 252, fat 19.6, fiber 7.8, carbs 13.1, protein 8.8

Tomato Cod Bake

Preparation time: 5 minutes

Cooking time: 12 minutes

Servings: 4

Ingredients:

• tablespoons butter, melted

• 2 tablespoons parsley, chopped

• ¼ cup keto tomato sauce 8 cherry tomatoes, halved

• 2 cod fillets, boneless, skinless and cubed Salt and black pepper to the taste

Directions:

2. In a baking pan that fits the air fryer, combine all the ingredients, toss, put the pan in the machine and cook the mix at 390 degrees F for 12 minutes. Divide the mix into bowls and serve for lunch.

Nutrition: calories 232, fat 8, fiber 2, carbs 5, protein 11

Wrapped Zucchini

Prep time: 10 minutes

Cooking time: 10 minutes

Servings: 2

Ingredients:

- 2 zucchinis, trimmed

- 8 bacon slices

- 1 teaspoon sesame oil

- ¼ teaspoon chili powder

Directions:

2.   Cut every zucchini into 4 sticks and sprinkle with chili powder. Then wrap every zucchini stick in bacon and sprinkle with sesame oil. Preheat the air fryer to 400F. Put the zucchini sticks in the air fryer in one layer and cook for 10 minutes. Flip the zucchini sticks after 5 minutes of cooking.

Nutrition: calories 464, fat 34.4, fiber 2.3, carbs 7.8, protein 30.6

Parsley Turkey Stew

Preparation time: 5 minutes

Cooking time: 25 minutes

Servings: 4

Ingredients:

•   1 turkey breast, skinless, boneless and cubed 1 tablespoon olive oil

•   1 broccoli head, florets separated 1 cup keto tomato sauce

•   Salt and black pepper to the taste 1 tablespoon parsley, chopped

Directions:

2.   In a baking dish that fits your air fryer, mix the turkey with the rest of the ingredients except the parsley, toss, introduce the dish in the fryer, bake at 380 degrees F for 25 minutes, divide into bowls, sprinkle the parsley on top and serve.

Nutrition: calories 250, fat 11, fiber 2, carbs 6, protein 12

Chicken, Eggs and Lettuce Salad

Prep time: 15 minutes

Cooking time: 8 minutes

Servings: 3

Ingredients:

- 3 spring onions, sliced
- 8 oz chicken fillet, roughly chopped
- 1 bacon slice, cooked, crumbled
- 2 cherry tomatoes, halved
- ¼ avocado, chopped
- 2 eggs, hard-boiled, peeled, chopped
- 1 cup lettuce, roughly chopped
- 1 tablespoon sesame oil
- ½ teaspoon lemon juice
- ½ teaspoon avocado oil
- ½ teaspoon ground black pepper
- ½ teaspoon salt
- 1 egg, beaten

- 2 tablespoons coconut flakes

Directions:

1.   Sprinkle the chopped chicken fillets with salt and ground black pepper. Then dip the chicken in the egg and after this, coat in the coconut flakes.

2.   Preheat the air fryer to 385F. Place the chicken fillets inside and sprinkle them with avocado oil. Cook the chicken pieces for 8 minutes. Shake them after 4 minutes of cooking. After this, in the mixing bowl mix up spring onions, bacon, cherry tomatoes, hard-boiled eggs, lettuce, and lemon juice.

3.   Add sesame oil and shake the salad well. When the chicken is cooked, add it in the cobb salad and mix up gently with the help of the wooden spatulas.

Nutrition: calories 355, fat 22.5, fiber 2.8, carbs 7.2, protein 31.1

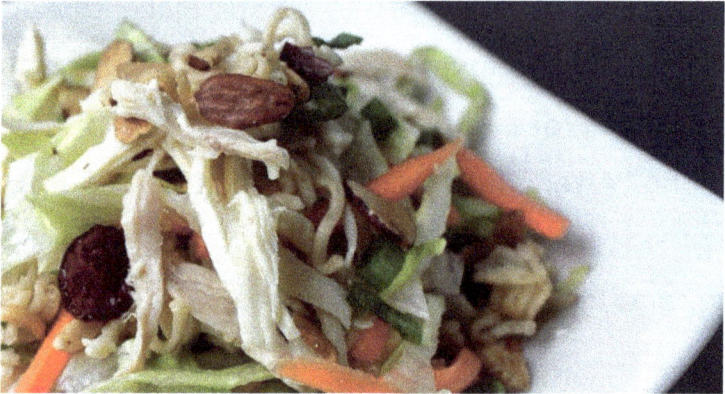

Pork and Spinach Stew

Preparation time: 5 minutes

Cooking time: 25 minutes

Servings: 4

Ingredients:

- 1 pound pork stew meat, cubed 3 garlic cloves, minced

- ¼ cup keto tomato sauce 1 cup spinach, torn

- ½ teaspoon olive oil

Directions:

1. In pan that fits your air fryer, mix the pork with the other ingredients except the spinach, toss, introduce in the fryer and cook at 370 degrees F for 15 minutes. Add the spinach, toss, cook for 10 minutes more, divide into bowls and serve for lunch.

Nutrition: calories 290, fat 14, fiber 3, carbs 5, protein 13

Chicken, Eggs and Lettuce Salad

Prep time: 15 minutes

Cooking time: 8 minutes

Servings: 3

Ingredients:

- 3 spring onions, sliced
- 8 oz chicken fillet, roughly chopped
- 1 bacon slice, cooked, crumbled
- 2 cherry tomatoes, halved
- ¼ avocado, chopped
- 2 eggs, hard-boiled, peeled, chopped
- 1 cup lettuce, roughly chopped
- 1 tablespoon sesame oil
- ½ teaspoon lemon juice
- ½ teaspoon avocado oil
- ½ teaspoon ground black pepper
- ½ teaspoon salt
- 1 egg, beaten

- 2 tablespoons coconut flakes

Directions:

1.   Sprinkle the chopped chicken fillets with salt and ground black pepper. Then dip the chicken in the egg and after this, coat in the coconut flakes. Preheat the air fryer to 385F.

2.   Place the chicken fillets inside and sprinkle them with avocado oil. Cook the chicken pieces for 8 minutes. Shake them after 4 minutes of cooking. After this, in the mixing bowl mix up spring onions, bacon, cherry tomatoes, hard-boiled eggs, lettuce, and lemon juice.

3.   Add sesame oil and shake the salad well. When the chicken is cooked, add it in the cobb salad and mix up gently with the help of the wooden spatulas.

Nutrition: calories 355, fat 22.5, fiber 2.8, carbs 7.2, protein 31.1

Pork and Spinach Stew

Preparation time: 5 minutes

Cooking time: 25 minutes

Servings: 4

Ingredients:

- 1 pound pork stew meat, cubed 3 garlic cloves, minced

- ¼ cup keto tomato sauce 1 cup spinach, torn

- ½ teaspoon olive oil

Directions:

2. In pan that fits your air fryer, mix the pork with the other ingredients except the spinach, toss, introduce in the fryer and cook at 370 degrees F for 15 minutes. Add the spinach, toss, cook for 10 minutes more, divide into bowls and serve for lunch.

Nutrition: calories 290, fat 14, fiber 3, carbs 5, protein 13

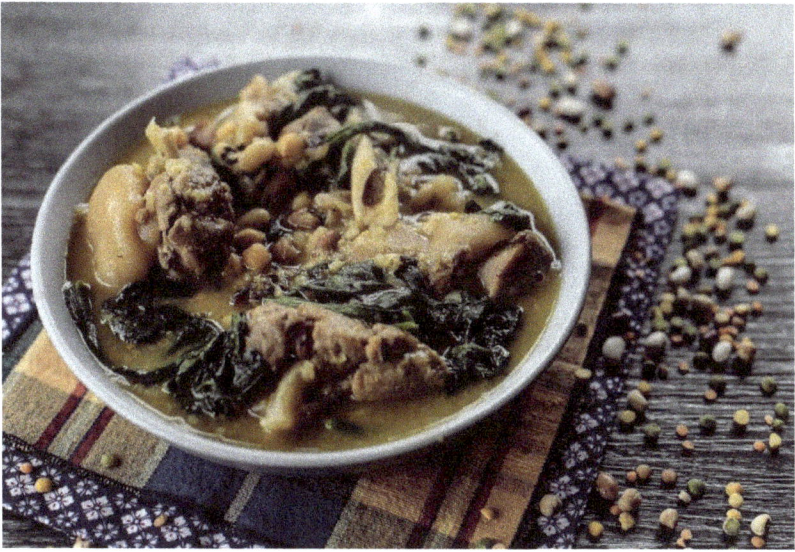

Pancetta Salad

Prep time: 10 minutes

Cooking time: 10 minutes

 Servings: 3

Ingredients:

- 2 cups iceberg lettuce, chopped

- 6 oz pancetta, chopped

- ½ teaspoon ground black pepper

- ½ teaspoon olive oil

- 3 oz Parmesan, grated

Directions:

1. Mix up pancetta, ground black pepper, and olive oil. Preheat the air fryer to 365F. Put the chopped pancetta in the air fryer and cook for 10 minutes Shake the pancetta every 3 minutes to avoid burning. Meanwhile, in the salad bowl combine iceberg lettuce with grated parmesan. Then add cooked pancetta and mix up the salad.

Nutrition: calories 410, fat 30.6, fiber 0.3, carbs 3.2, protein 30.3

Mustard Chicken

Preparation time: 5 minutes

Cooking time: 30 minutes

Servings: 4

Ingredients:

- and ½ pounds chicken thighs, bone-in 2 tablespoons Dijon mustard

- A pinch of salt and black pepper Cooking spray

Directions:

1. In a bowl, mix the chicken thighs with all the other ingredients and toss. Put the chicken in your Air Fryer's basket and cook at 370 degrees F for 30 minutes shaking halfway. Serve these chicken thighs for lunch.

Nutrition: calories 253, fat 17, fiber 3, carbs 6, protein 12

Lemon Chicken Mix

Prep time: 15 minutes

Cooking time: 15 minutes

Servings: 3

Ingredients:

- 4 chicken thighs, skinless, boneless

- 1 tablespoon lemon juice

- 1 teaspoon ground paprika

- ½ teaspoon salt

- ½ teaspoon ground black pepper

- 1 tablespoon sesame oil

- ½ teaspoon dried parsley

- ½ teaspoon keto tomato sauce

Directions:

1. Cut the chicken thighs into halves and put them in the bowl. Add lemon juice, ground paprika, salt, ground black pepper, sesame oil, parsley, and tomato sauce. Mix up the chicken with the help of the fingertips and leave

for 10-15 minutes to marinate. Then string the meat on the wooden skewers and put in the preheated to 375F air fryer. Cook the tavuk shish for 10 minutes at 375F. Then flip the meal on another side and cook for 5 minutes more.

Nutrition: calories 415, fat 19.1, fiber 0.4, carbs 0.9, protein 56.6

Stuffed Avocado

Prep time: 15 minutes

Cooking time: 10 minutes

Servings: 2

Ingredients:

- 1 avocado, peeled, pitted
- 2 tablespoons coconut flour
- 1 egg, beaten
- 1 tablespoon pork rinds, grinded
- 1 oz ground pork
- 1 oz Parmesan, grated
- 1 teaspoon avocado oil
- Cooking spray

Directions:

1.   Heat up the skillet on the medium heat and add avocado oil. Add ground pork and cook it for 3 minutes. Stir it from time to time to avoid burning. Then add grated cheese and stir the mixture until cheese is melted.

2. Remove the mixture from the heat. After this, fill the avocado with the ground pork mixture and pork rinds. Secure two halves of avocado together and dip in the egg. Then coat the avocado in the coconut four and dip in the egg again. After this, coat the avocado in the coconut flour one more time. Preheat the air fryer to 400F. Place the avocado bomb in the air fryer and spray it with cooking spray. Cook the meal for 6 minutes at 400F. Cut the cooked avocado bomb into 2 servings and transfer in the serving plate.

Nutrition: calories 398, fat 31.4, fiber 9.7, carbs 13.8, protein 18.9

Almond Sea Bream

Prep time: 15 minutes

Cooking time: 10 minutes

Servings: 3

Ingredients:

- 1-pound sea bream steaks (pieces)

- 1 egg, beaten

- 1 tablespoon coconut flour

- 1 teaspoon garlic powder

- 1 tablespoon almond butter, melted

- ½ teaspoon Erythritol

- ½ teaspoon chili powder

- 1 teaspoon apple cider vinegar

Directions:

1.   In the shallow bowl mix up garlic powder, coconut flour, chili powder, and Erythritol. Sprinkle the sea bream steaks with apple cider vinegar and dip in the beaten egg. After this, coat every fish steak in the coconut flour

mixture. Preheat the air fryer to 390F. Place the fish steak in the air fryer in one layer and sprinkle with almond butter. Cook them for 5 minutes from each side.

Nutrition: calories 273, fat 9.9, fiber 1.6, carbs 3.4, protein 39.8

Coconut Flounder

Preparation time: 5 minutes

Cooking time: 12 minutes

Servings: 2

Ingredients:

- 2 flounder fillets, boneless 2 garlic cloves, minced

- 2 teaspoons coconut aminos 2 tablespoons lemon juice

- A pinch of salt and black pepper

- ½ teaspoon stevia

- 2 tablespoons olive oil

Directions:

1. In a pan that fits your air fryer, mix all the ingredients, toss, introduce in the fryer and cook at 390 degrees F for 12 minutes. Divide into bowls and serve.

Nutrition: calories 251, fat 13, fiber 3, carbs 5, protein 10

Paprika Prawns

Prep time: 15 minutes

Cooking time: 5 minutes

Servings: 5

Ingredients:

- 3-pound prawns, peeled

- 1 tablespoon ground turmeric

- 1 teaspoon smoked paprika

- 1 tablespoon coconut milk

- 1 teaspoon avocado oil

- ½ teaspoon salt

Directions:

1.   Put the prawns in the bowl and sprinkle them with ground turmeric, smoked paprika, and salt. Then add coconut milk and leave them for 10 minutes to marinate. Meanwhile, preheat the air fryer to 400F. Put the marinated prawns in the air fryer basket and sprinkle

with avocado oil. Cook the prawns for 3 minutes. Then shake them well and cook for 2 minutes more.

Nutrition: calories 338, fat 5.6, fiber 0.6, carbs 5.5, protein 62.2

Flounder with Ginger Mushrooms

Preparation time: 5 minutes

Cooking time: 15 minutes

Servings: 4

Ingredients:

- 4 flounder fillets, boneless
- 2 tablespoons coconut aminos A pinch of salt and black pepper
- and ½ teaspoons ginger, grated 2 teaspoons olive oil
- green onions, chopped 2 cups mushrooms, sliced

Directions:

1. Heat u a pan that fits your air fryer with the oil over medium-high heat, add the mushrooms and all the other ingredients except the fish, toss and sauté for 5 minutes. Add the fish, toss gently, introduce the pan in the fryer and cook at 390 degrees F for 10 minutes. Divide between plates and serve.

Nutrition: calories 271, fat 12, fiber 4, carbs 6, protein 11

Cobbler

Prep time: 15 minutes

Cooking time: 30 minutes

Servings: 4

Ingredients:

- ¼ cup heavy cream

- 1 egg, beaten

- ½ cup almond flour

- 1 teaspoon vanilla extract

- 2 tablespoons butter, softened

- ¼ cup hazelnuts, chopped

Directions:

1.   Mix up heavy cream, egg, almond flour, vanilla extract, and   butter. Then whisk the mixture gently. Preheat the air fryer to 325F. Line the air fryer pan with baking paper. Pour ½ part of the batter in the baking pan, flatten it gently and top with hazelnuts. Then pour

the remaining batter over the hazelnuts and place the pan in the air fryer. Cook the cobbler for 30 minutes.

Nutrition: calories 145, fat 14.2, fiber 0.8, carbs 2, protein 3

Lemon and Thyme Sea bass

Prep time: 10 minutes

Cooking time: 15 minutes

Servings: 3

Ingredients:

- 8 oz sea bass, trimmed, peeled

- 4 lemon slices

- 1 tablespoon thyme

- 2 teaspoons sesame oil

- 1 teaspoon salt

Directions:

1.   Fill the sea bass with lemon slices and rub with thyme, salt, and sesame oil. Then preheat the air fryer to 385F and put the fish in the air fryer basket. Cook it for 12 minutes. Then flip the fish on another side and cook it for 3 minutes more.

Nutrition: calories 216, fat 7.9, fiber 0.6, carbs 6.3, protein 0.2

Buttery Chives Trout

Preparation time: 10 minutes

Cooking time: 12 minutes

Servings: 4

Ingredients:

• 4 trout fillets, boneless

• 4 tablespoons butter, melted

• Salt and black pepper to the taste Juice of 1 lime

• tablespoon chives, chopped 1 tablespoon parsley, chopped

Directions:

1. Mix the fish fillets with the melted butter, salt and pepper, rub gently, put the fish in your air fryer's basket and cook at 390 degrees F for 6 minutes on each side. Divide between plates and serve with lime juice drizzled on top and with parsley and chives sprinkled at the end.

Nutrition: calories 221, fat 11, fiber 4, carbs 6, protein 9

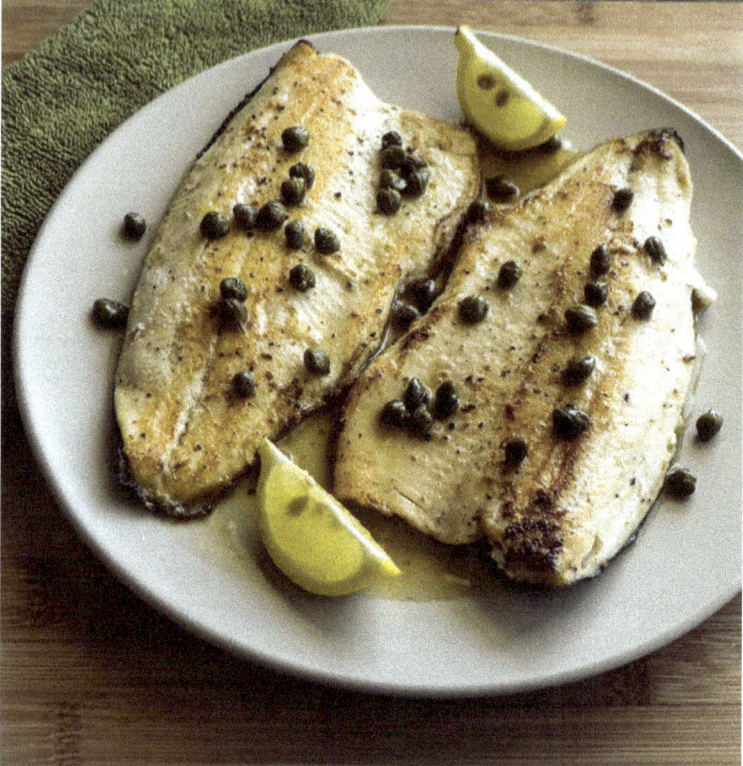

Italian Halibut and Asparagus

Prep time: 10 minutes

Cooking time: 7 minutes

Servings: 2

Ingredients:

- 2 halibut fillets
- 4 oz asparagus, trimmed
- 1 tablespoon avocado oil
- ½ teaspoon garlic powder
- 1 teaspoon Italian seasonings
- 1 teaspoon butter
- 1 teaspoon salt
- 1 tablespoon lemon juice

Directions:

1. Chop the halibut fillet roughly and sprinkle with garlic powder and Italian seasonings. Preheat the air fryer to 400F. Put the asparagus in the air fryer basket and sprinkle it with salt. Then put the fish over the

asparagus and sprinkle it with avocado oil and lemon juice. Cook the meal for 8 minutes. Then transfer it in the serving plates and top with butter.

Nutrition: calories 367, fat 10.3, fiber 1.6, carbs 3.5, protein 62.1

Parmesan and Garlic Trout

Preparation time: 5 minutes

Cooking time: 15 minutes

Servings: 4

Ingredients:

• tablespoons olive oil 2 garlic cloves, minced

• ½ cup chicken stock

• Salt and black pepper to the taste 4 trout fillets, boneless

• ¾ cup parmesan, grated

• ¼ cup tarragon, chopped

Directions:

1. In a pan that fits your air fryer, mix all the ingredients except the fish and the parmesan and whisk. Add the fish and grease it well with this mix.

2. Sprinkle the parmesan on top, put the pan in the air fryer and cook at 380 degrees F for 15 minutes. Divide everything between plates and serve.

Nutrition: calories 271, fat 12, fiber 4, carbs 6, protein 11

Italian Mackerel

Prep time: 20 minutes

Cooking time: 15 minutes

Servings: 2

Ingredients:

- 8 oz mackerel, trimmed
- 1 tablespoon Italian seasonings
- 1 teaspoon keto tomato sauce
- 2 tablespoons ghee, melted
- ½ teaspoon salt

Directions:

1.   Rub the mackerel with Italian seasonings, and tomato sauce. After this, rub the fish with salt and leave for 15 minutes in the fridge to marinate. Meanwhile, preheat the air fryer to 390F. When the time of marinating is finished, brush the fish with ghee and wrap in the baking paper. Place the wrapped fish in the air fryer and cook it for 15 minutes.

Nutrition: calories 433, fat 35, fiber 0.1, carbs 1.3, protein 27.2

Salmon Skewers

Prep time: 15 minutes

Cooking time: 10 minutes

Servings: 4

Ingredients:

• 1-pound salmon fillet

• 4 oz bacon, sliced

• 2 mozzarella balls, sliced

• ½ teaspoon avocado oil

• ½ teaspoon chili flakes

Directions:

1. Cut the salmon into the medium size cubes (4 cubes per serving) Then sprinkle salmon cubes with chili flakes and wrap in the sliced bacon.

2. String the wrapped salmon cubes on the skewers and sprinkle with avocado oil. After this, preheat the air fryer to 400F. Put the salmon skewers in the preheat air fryer basket and cook them at 400F for 4 minutes. Then

flip the skewers on another side and cook them for 6 minutes at 385F.

Nutrition: calories 364, fat 23.4, fiber 0, carbs 0.5, protein 37.5

Green Beans Stew

Preparation time: 5 minutes

Cooking time: 15 minutes

Servings: 4

Ingredients:

•   1 pound green beans, halved 1 cup okra

•   1 tablespoon thyme, chopped

•   3 tablespoons keto tomato sauce Salt and black pepper to the taste 4 garlic cloves, minced

Directions:

1.   In a pan that fits your air fryer, mix all the ingredients, toss, introduce the pan in the air fryer and cook at 370 degrees F for 15 minutes. Divide the stew into bowls and serve.

Nutrition: calories 183, fat 5, fiber 2, carbs 4, protein 8

Beef and Green Onions Casserole

Prep time: 15 minutes

Cooking time: 21 minutes

Servings: 4

Ingredients:

- 10 oz lean ground beef

- 1 oz green onions, chopped

- 2 low carb tortillas

- 1 cup Mexican cheese blend, shredded

- 1 teaspoon fresh cilantro, chopped

- 1 teaspoon butter

- 1 tablespoon mascarpone

- 1 tablespoon heavy cream

- ¼ teaspoon garlic powder

- 1 teaspoon Mexican seasonings

- 1 teaspoon olive oil

Directions:

1.   Pour olive oil in the skillet and heat it up over the medium heat. Then add ground beef and sprinkle it with garlic powder and Mexican seasonings. Cook the ground beef for 7 minutes over the medium heat. Stir it from time to time Then chop the low carb tortillas. Grease the air fryer pan with butter and put the tortillas in one layer inside. Put the ground beef mixture over the tortillas and spread it gently with the help of the spoon. Then sprinkle it with cilantro, green onions, mascarpone, and heavy cream. Top the casserole with Mexican cheese blend and cover with baking paper.

2.   Secure the edges of the pan well. Preheat the air fryer to 360F. Cook the casserole for 10 minutes at 360F and then remove the baking paper and cook the meal for 5 minutes more to reach the crunchy crust.

Nutrition: calories 179, fat 14.7, fiber 3, carbs 6.6, protein 23.8

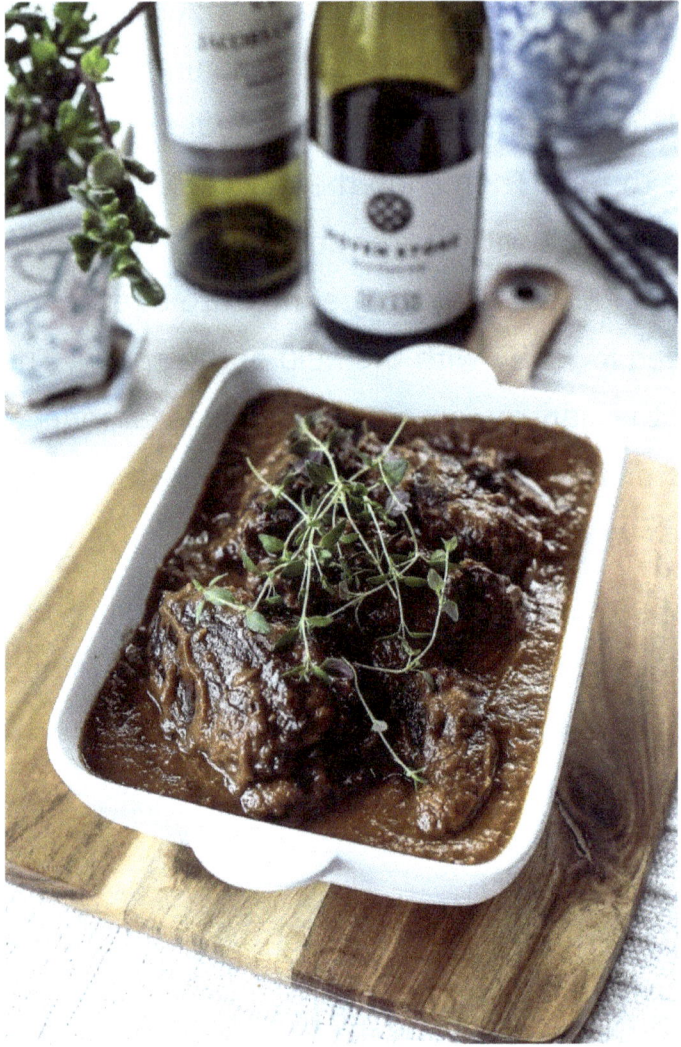

Rosemary Chicken Stew

Preparation time: 5 minutes

Cooking time: 20 minutes

Servings: 4

Ingredients:

• 2 cups okra

• 2 garlic cloves, minced

• 1 pound chicken breasts, skinless, boneless and cubed 4 tomatoes, cubed

• 1 tablespoon olive oil

• teaspoon rosemary, dried

• Salt and black pepper to the taste 1 tablespoon parsley, chopped

Directions:

1.   Heat up a pan that fits your air fryer with the oil over medium-high heat, add the chicken, garlic, rosemary, salt and pepper, toss and brown for 5 minutes. Add the remaining ingredients, toss again, place the pan

in the air fryer and cook at 380 degrees F for 15 minutes more. Divide the stew into bowls and serve for lunch.

Nutrition: calories 220, fat 13, fiber 3, carbs 5, protein 11

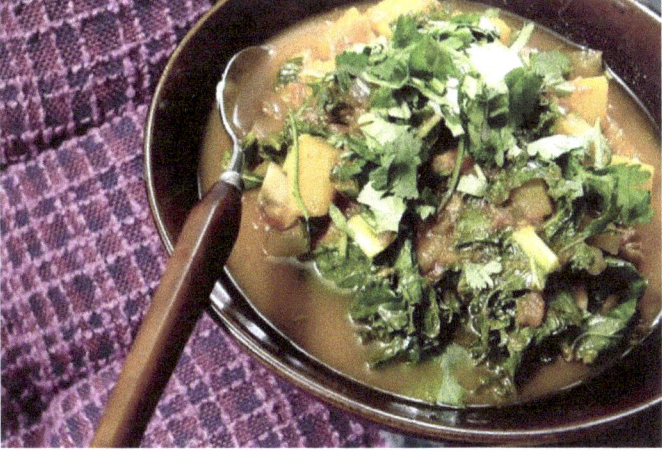

Cheese Quiche

Prep time: 20 minutes

Cooking time: 19 minutes

Servings: 5

Ingredients:

- ½ cup almond flour
- 1 tablespoon Psyllium husk
- ½ teaspoon flax meal
- ¼ teaspoon baking powder
- 2 eggs, beaten
- 7 oz Feta cheese, crumbled
- ¼ cup scallions, diced
- ½ teaspoon ground black pepper
- ¼ teaspoon ground cardamom
- 1 oz Parmesan, grated
- 1 teaspoon coconut oil, melted
- 3 tablespoons almond butter

Directions:

1.   Make the quiche crust: mix up almond flour, Psyllium husk, flax meal, baking powder, and almond butter in the bowl. Stir the mixture until homogenous and knead the non-sticky dough. Then pour melted coconut oil in the skillet and bring it to boil. Add scallions and cook it for 3 minutes or until it is light brown.

2.   Then transfer the cooked onion in the mixing bowl. Add Parmesan, ground cardamom, and ground black pepper. After this, add Feta cheese and eggs. Stir the mass until homogenous. Cut the dough into 5 pieces. Place the dough in the quiche molds and flatten it in the shape of the pie crust with the help of the fingertips.

3.   Then fill every quiche crust with a Feta mixture. Preheat the air fryer to 365F. Put the molds with quiche in the air fryer basket and cook them for 15 minutes.

Nutrition: calories 254, fat 19.2, fiber 7.3, carbs 12.5, protein 12.5

Spring Onions and Shrimp Mix

Preparation time: 5 minutes

Cooking time: 15 minutes

Servings: 4

Ingredients:

* cups baby spinach

* ¼ cup veggie stock 2 tomatoes, cubed

* 1 tablespoon garlic, minced

* 15 ounces shrimp, peeled and deveined 4 spring onions, chopped

* ½ teaspoon cumin, ground 1 tablespoon lemon juice

* 2 tablespoons cilantro, chopped Salt and black pepper to the taste

Directions:

1. In a pan that fits your air fryer, mix all the ingredients except the cilantro, toss, introduce in the air

fryer and cook at 360 degrees F for 15 minutes. Add the cilantro, stir, divide into bowls and serve for lunch.

Nutrition: calories 201, fat 8, fiber 2, carbs 4, protein 8

Chili Sloppy Joes

Prep time: 10 minutes

Cooking time: 20 minutes

Servings: 3

Ingredients:

- 1 cup ground pork
- 1 teaspoon sloppy Joes seasonings
- 1 teaspoon butter
- 1 tablespoon keto tomato sauce
- 1 teaspoon mustard
- ¼ cup beef broth
- ½ teaspoon chili flakes
- ½ bell pepper, chopped
- ½ teaspoon minced garlic

Directions:

1.   In the bowl mix up chili flakes, beef broth, minced garlic, and tomato sauce. Add mustard and whisk the

liquid until homogenous. After this, add ground pork and sloppy Joes seasonings. Stir the ingredients with the help of the spoon and transfer in the air fryer baking pan. Add butter.

2.   Preheat the air fryer to 365F. Put the pan with sloppy Joe in the air fryer basket and cook the meal for 20 minutes. Stir the meal well after 10 minutes of cooking.

Nutrition: calories 344, fat 23.4, fiber 0.2, carbs 3.4, protein 27.8

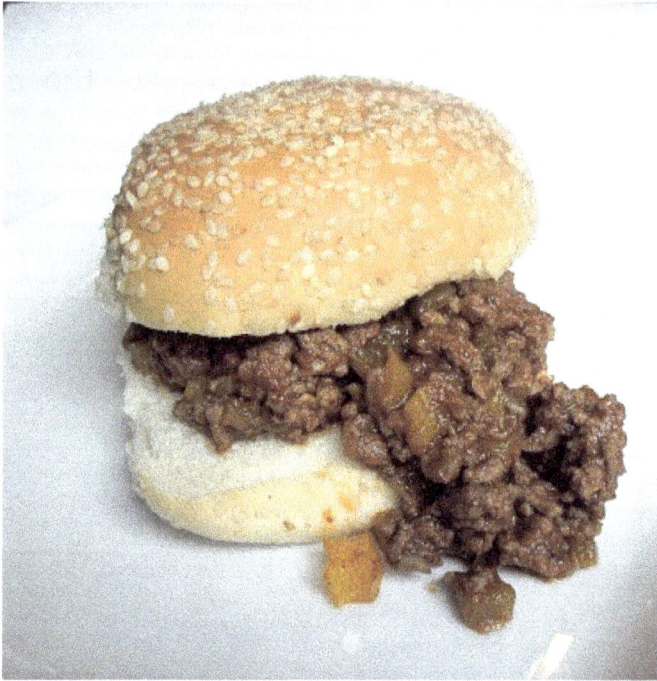

Tomato and Peppers Stew

Preparation time: 5 minutes

Cooking time: 15 minutes

Servings: 4

Ingredients:

- 4 spring onions, chopped 2 pound tormatoes, cubed 1 teaspoon sweet paprika

- Salt and black pepper to the taste 2 red bell peppers, cubed

- tablespoon cilantro, chopped

Directions:

1. In a pan that fits your air fryer, mix all the ingredients, toss, introduce the pan in the fryer and cook at 360 degrees F for 15 minutes. Divide into bowls and serve for lunch.

Nutrition: calories 185, fat 3, fiber 2, carbs 4, protein 9

Tuna Bake

Prep time: 15 minutes

Cooking time: 15 minutes

Servings: 6

Ingredients:

- 2 spring onions, diced
- 1 pound smoked tuna, boneless
- ¼ cup ricotta cheese
- 3 oz celery stalk, diced
- ½ teaspoon celery seeds
- 1 tablespoon cream cheese
- ¼ teaspoon salt
- ½ teaspoon ground paprika
- 2 tablespoons lemon juice
- 1 tablespoon ghee
- 4 oz Edam cheese, shredded

Directions:

1.   Mix up celery seeds, cream cheese, ground paprika, lemon juice, and ricotta cheese. Then shred the tuna until it is smooth and add it in the cream cheese mixture. Add onion and stir the mass with the help of the spoon. Grease the air fryer pan with ghee and put the tuna mixture inside. Flatten its surface gently with the help of the spoon and top with Edam cheese. Preheat the air fryer to 360F. Place the pan with tuna melt in the air fryer and cook it for 15 minutes.

Nutrition: calories 249, fat 14.3, fiber 1.1, carbs 5, protein 24.2

Fennel Stew

Preparation time: 5 minutes

Cooking time: 15 minutes

Servings: 4

Ingredients:

- cups tomatoes, cubed 2 fennel bulbs, shredded

- ½ cup chicken stock

- 2 tablespoons keto tomato puree 1 red bell pepper, chopped

- 2 garlic cloves, minced

- 1 teaspoon sweet paprika 1 teaspoon rosemary, dried

- Salt and black pepper to the taste

Directions:

2.   In a pan that fits your air fryer, mix all the ingredients, toss, introduce in the fryer and cook at 380 degrees F for 15 minutes. Divide the stew into bowls and serve for lunch.

Nutrition: calories 184, fat 7, fiber 2, carbs 3, protein 8

www.ingramcontent.com/pod-product-compliance
Lightning Source LLC
Chambersburg PA
CBHW050756030426
42336CB00012B/1841